W9-AMT-300

The 2003 Pfizer Medical School Manual

A Practical Guide to Getting into
Medical School

Mike Magee, MD

Library of Congress Cataloguing-in-Publication Data
Magee, Mike
The 2003 Pfizer Medical School Manual/Mike Magee, MD
104 p.   1 cm.
1. Magee, Mike
2. Education Higher-United States
3. Directories
I. Title
L901.C33.1996   378.73   96-47529
ISBN: 1-889793-06-X
Printed in Canada

The 2003 Pfizer Medical School Manual
is provided as part of the
Pfizer Medical Humanities Initiative,

a program which encourages
the development of humanistically
and scientifically balanced
physicians committed to
patients, families, and
their communities.

For more information about the
Pfizer Medical Humanities Initiative,
contact:
http://www.positiveprofiles.com

Table of Contents

I
Introduction

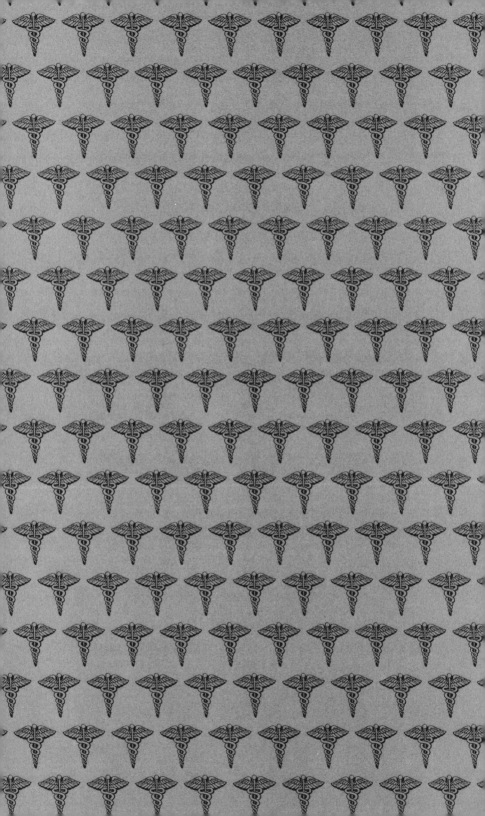

An Introductory Message by Author
Mike Magee, MD

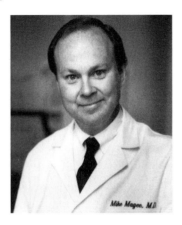

Mike Magee, M.D.

*T*his book is dedicated to those who seek to devote their lives to a career in medicine. It is intended to assist would-be physicians as they navigate the complex and often daunting medical school admissions process.

In an era that heralds accelerated breakthroughs and scientific discoveries, medical science is on the brink of an unprecedented ability to understand and manipulate human life. Our understanding of the genetic and molecular mechanisms underlying diseases has greatly expanded the scope of the possible. Knowledge of the genome will allow us to predict and prevent diseases before they start. Future physicians can anticipate a constant stream of newly minted medical advances to revolutionize their medical practice, particularly the treatment of heart disease, arthritis, diabetes, Alzheimer's and cancer.

Physicians who thoughtfully and passionately embrace this medical and technological revolution will shape the future of medicine. Medicine will also be shaped by demographic changes. By 2030, 50 percent of American adults will be 50 or more years old, and the population of adults over 85 years old will have doubled. The challenge of meeting the ever-increasing *demand for quality health care will depend upon progress in scientific understanding.*

Through all the medical breakthroughs and demographic changes to come, our need for interpersonal connection will remain. Medicine will always be a profession that marries the role of medical mystery solver with compassionate healer. Medical schools will forever seek students who communicate effectively, who rigorously pursue intellectual excellence, and who find purpose, satisfaction and dignity in human service.

This book is not a secret formula that will guarantee admission to medical school. It does provide aspiring physicians with specific, practical recommendations that will help them positively and memorably present themselves to prospective medical schools. With a call to those committed to transforming their knowledge of health and science into actions that will improve people's lives, and with wholehearted endorsement of your career choice, I urge tomorrow's physicians onward!

Sincerely,

Mike Magee ms

Mike Magee, MD

II
Overview

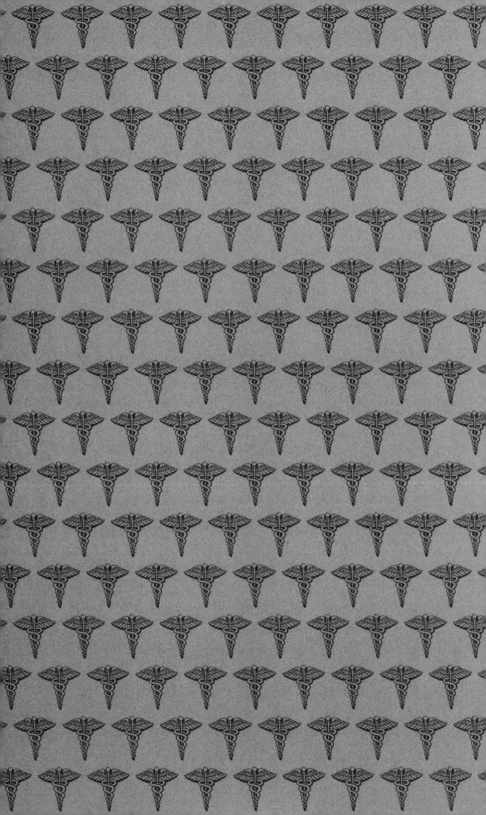

II Overview

There are approximately 80,000 students at any one time enrolled in America's 144 medical schools. Each year this unique body of talented and diverse individuals is revitalized with approximately 19,500 women and men chosen from more than 48,500 applicants. These medical students are highly qualified, having fulfilled exacting science requirements and achieved excellent grade point averages and MCAT scores.

With more than twice as many applicants as there are seats, how do medical schools decide whom to accept? Four criteria are used to evaluate applicants:
- Grade point average, 25%
- MCAT scores, 25%
- Letters of recommendation, 25%
- Interviews, 25% and often the determining factor in accepting or rejecting candidates.

As important as the interview is, preparation for it is often overlooked. The rigorous undergraduate science curriculum, the demanding process of choosing and applying to schools, the hours of study for MCAT exams, and the development of relationships with professors who will write insightful, personal letters of recommendation often take precedence over preparation for an admissions interview. Yet, successful interviews require research, introspection and analytical thought. Chapter IV of this manual prepares applicants for medical school interviews.

Undergraduate Preparation

Today, medical schools accept a broad range of undergraduate majors. Indeed, approximately 15% of the medical school Class of 2005 (who entered medical school in Fall, 2001) majored in liberal arts. Fully 42% of liberal arts applicants for the Class of 2005 were accepted into medical school, coming close to the overall acceptance rate of 50%. Still, most applicants choose a traditional path, with approximately 70% of the medical school Class of 2005 majoring in biological or physical sciences.

Most colleges and universities maintain a pre-medical advisory office. While advice on curriculum choices varies from school to school, undergraduates should enroll in courses that will develop their competence in required sciences as well as contribute to their well-rounded candidacy.

Most medical schools require successful completion of the following laboratory courses:
- introductory biology (one year)
- inorganic or general chemistry (one year)
- organic chemistry (one year)
- physics (one year)

Other courses commonly required include:
- calculus or college math
- English (one year)
- humanities electives

- anatomy and physiology
- biochemistry
- genetics

Since the MCAT test required for admission to medical school assesses your knowledge of science concepts and principles, as well as problem-solving, critical thinking and writing skills, complete these courses during the first three years of college so that by your junior year you can take the April or August MCATs.

Allopathic vs. Osteopathic Medical Schools

In the United States and its territories, 125 allopathic medical schools grant Doctorates of Medicine, or MDs, and 19 osteopathic medical schools grant Doctorates of Osteopathy, or D.O.s.

The first school of medicine in the United States was founded at the University of Pennsylvania in 1765 by John Morgan, a young surgeon. In 1892, some 127 years later, Andrew Taylor Still, MD, founded the first School of Osteopathic Medicine in Missouri. This school emphasized musculoskeletal training and manipulation to aid bodily function. Though chartered by state law to grant graduates an MD, Taylor chose instead to grant Doctorates of Osteopathy, or D.O.s.

Over the next century, the two branches of medicine often clashed. By 1974, the federal and state government as well as the American Medical Association recognized both MDs and D.O.s as legally separate but equal branches of medicine. Today, allopathic and osteopathic medical schools share the following characteristics:

- Applicants possess four-year undergraduate degrees and meet similar science prerequisites

- Accepted students must complete four years of medical school, including two years of didactic and two years of clinical experience

- Students may pursue specialist or generalist tracks

- Students must pass board exams for licensure

- Graduates are qualified to commence practice in fully accredited hospitals

To learn how the Class of 2006 enrolled in allopathic schools compared to the Class of 2006 enrolled in osteopathic schools, see Chapter V, pages 55-56. To learn more about allopathic medical schools, contact the Association of American Medical Colleges at (202) 828-0400. For osteopathic medical schools, contact the American Association of Colleges of Osteopathic Medicine at (301) 968-4100.

Application to Medical School

One hundred fifteen of the 125 allopathic medical schools and programs participate in the American Medical College Application Service, or AMCAS. The AMCAS electronic application is available on the web in April of each year. AMCAS processes and forwards your application and MCAT scores to the individual schools to which you apply beginning June 1st. Application through AMCAS allows you to complete the application process once and to simultaneously apply to any of the 115 participating allopathic schools. The 11 non-AMCAS allopathic medical schools are noted in Chapter VI.

The AMCAS application fee is based upon the number of schools to which applicants apply. The fee for an application is $150 for the first school and $30.00 for each additional school regardless of the point at which you add school designations. In addition to this fee, individual medical schools have application fees that range from $25 to $100. Upon receipt of your AMCAS application, each school usually sends secondary application materials as well as a bill for the school's individual application fee. Failure to remit this fee may result in no further action being taken on your application.

To obtain an AMCAS web application (the paper version is no longer produced) or additional information

about AMCAS, contact:
AMCAS
American Medical College Application Service
Section for Student Services
2501 M Street, NW, Lobby-26
Washington, DC 20037-1300
(202) 828-0600
www.aamc.org

All osteopathic medical schools participate in a comparable application service. The American Association of Colleges of Osteopathic Medicine Application Service, or AACOMAS, processes and forwards your application and MCAT scores to the individual schools to which you apply beginning June 1st.

To obtain an AACOMAS application, available in April, contact your college advisory office, AACOMAS participating schools, or AACOMAS at:
AACOMAS
American Association of Colleges of Osteopathic Medicine Application Service
5550 Friendship Blvd.
Suite 310
Chevy Chase, MD 20815
(301) 968-4190
www.aacom.org

The MCAT

The MCAT is a standardized multiple choice and written examination administered semi-annually, on an April Saturday and on an August Saturday. Most schools recommend that the test, which is required for admission to medical school, be taken 18 months before students submit their medical school applications. An April MCAT is recommended so that results are ready in time for your AMCAS and/or AACOMAS applications. While you may repeat the test, it is unwise to take MCATs "just for practice" because all MCAT scores are recorded on your application. It is best to do well on your first take.

The MCAT assesses problem-solving, critical thinking, writing skills and knowledge of science concepts and principles prerequisite to the study of medicine. The four components of the MCAT are:

- Verbal Reasoning, 60 questions, 85 minutes, a test of reading comprehension, reasoning skills and critical thought. Content is drawn from humanities, social sciences and natural sciences.

- Biological Sciences, 77 questions, 100 minutes, a test of general biology concepts and problem-solving skills that includes graphs, tables and charts.

- Physical Sciences, 77 questions, 100 minutes, a

test of physics, organic and inorganic chemistry, DNA and genetics concepts and problem-solving skills that includes graphs, tables and charts.

- Writing Sample, two essay questions, 60 minutes, a test of writing and analytical skills.

Four scores are reported, one for each section. Verbal Reasoning, Physical Sciences and Biological Sciences grades are scored on a scale from 1 (lowest) to 15 (highest). The Writing Sample is scored on a scale ranging from J (lowest) to T (highest).

Information and application for the April MCAT exam is generally available in February and can be obtained from your college advisory office or by contacting:

MCAT Program
P.O. Box 4056
Iowa City, IA 52243-4056
(319) 337-1357
www.aamc.org

Payment of approximately $180 covers administration of the MCAT exam and release of your test scores to AMCAS participation schools and 6 non-AMCAS participating schools The $180 MCAT fee may be reduced or waived. For waiver materials, contact the Association of American Medical Colleges at (202) 828-0416 or www.aamc.org.

In addition to test preparation texts such as Arco's, Flower's, Baron's, Gruber's Shaum's, Monarch's and Barnes and Noble's, students may find the following resources useful in preparing for the MCAT:

1. Association of American Medical Colleges
   MCAT Publication – Student Manual
   Membership and Publication Orders
   2450 N Street, NW
   Washington, DC 20037-1129
   (202) 828-0416
   www.aamc.org
   AAMC provides a student manual of sample tests and a tutorial video cassette.

2. Kaplan Educational Centers
   131 West 56th Street
   New York, NY 10019
   (800) KAP-TEST
   www.kaplan.com
   An MCAT review course is available.

3. Princeton Review
   2315 Broadway
   New York, NY 10024
   (212) 874-8282
   www.review.com
   An MCAT review course is available.

Early Decision Program

Ninety percent of American medical schools participate in an Early Decision Program for highly qualified applicants with a strong preference for one school. Students who enroll in this program agree to apply to no other school prior to the medical college's October 1 decision. Students agree to enroll in the early decision school if accepted. Students not accepted early decision may be deferred for consideration with regular candidates, or rejected.

One disadvantage of the EDP is that it prevents application to other schools until after October 1st. This delay can significantly decrease your chances of admission compared to an application submitted earlier in the cycle. In 2001, 67% of the 1,063 Early Decision Program candidates received acceptances. This is higher than the prior year's 60% acceptance rate for EDP candidates.

Recommended Number of Applications

For the Class of 2006, students applying to allopathic medical schools submitted an average of 11.6 applications. Students applying to osteopathic medical schools submitted applications to an average of 5.7 medical schools.

The data indicates little difference in acceptance rates for those applying to multiple schools. In 2000, those who applied to seven to nineteen allopathic schools were accepted by 46% of the schools to which they applied, while those who applied to more than twenty schools had an acceptance rate of 53.1%. More important than acceptance rates is choosing schools that match your specific qualifications and interests, and that have historically accepted students from your college.

A number of factors may enhance your chances for admission. These include state residency, institutions where you apply early decision or have an existing personal connection, and membership in a special interest group.

Selecting a Medical School

To decide upon a medical school, read available literature both from and about different schools, visit campuses and their web sites, and discuss schools with your advisors and with current medical students. 10 factors to consider when comparing schools are:

1. Policies favoring state residents
2. Size of student body
3. Student:faculty ratio
4. Patient contact opportunities
5. Geographic location
6. Student services
7. Sources of financial support
8. Cost
9. Unique volunteer/research/leadership activities

10. Post graduate study opportunities

Differences in curriculum should also be noted. 10 curricular areas expanding in American medical schools are:
1. Nutrition
2. Geriatrics
3. Epidemiology
4. Environmental health
5. Preventive health care
6. Medical humanities
7. Medical ethics
8. Clinical decision making
9. Medical information systems
10. Socioeconomics of medicine

Chances for admission may be enhanced if the following characteristics apply to you:
1. State resident
2. Woman
3. Under-represented minority
4. Willingness to practice in under-served or rural areas
5. Plans to become a primary care physician
6. Relationship with alumni member
7. Residence in adjacent, contractually linked states
8. Early submission of application
9. Your college is one of the medical school's "feeder" schools
10. Credentials comparable to or exceeding the school's applicant pool

III

The Application Process

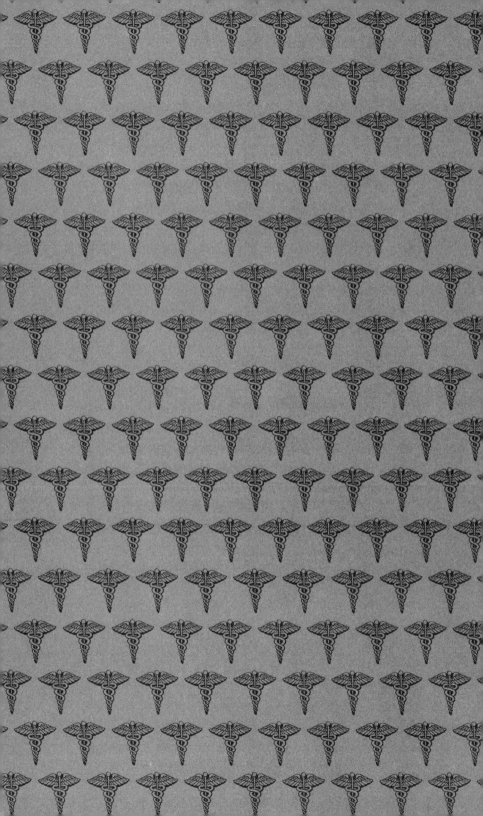

III The Application Process

Calendar of Deadlines

Entering Medical School in 2004

MCAT Review/Applications	January, 2003
April MCAT Registration	February 1, 2003
April MCAT Registration Deadline	March 28, 2003
AMCAS Begin Accepting Official Transcripts	March 15, 2003
AACOMAS Begin Accepting Official Transcripts	April 1, 2003
April MCAT Administered	April 26, 2003
AACOMAS Paper and Web Application Available	May 1, 2003
AMCAS Web Application Available	April, 2003
AMCAS Submissions Begin	April, 2003
AACOMAS Submissions Begin	Anytime after application is available
April MCAT Results Available	June 20, 2003
August MCAT Registration Deadline	July 12, 2003
Optimal Submission of Complete Application	July, 2003
Early Decision Program Application Filed	August 1, 2003
Early Decision Application Complete	August 1, 2003
August MCAT Administered	August 16, 2003
Early Decision Rendered	October 1, 2003
August MCAT Results Available	October 18, 2003
Application Deadline for Most Medical Schools	November 1, 2003

Timeline

Create a timeline by first deciding when you want to enter medical school. Then, in sequential order, follow these steps:

1. Fulfill science requirements

Basic undergraduate sciences in biology, chemistry and physics, including laboratories, are a prerequisite for application to medical school. To be competitive, you should attain A's and B's in these courses. By January of your junior year, request and verify the accuracy of transcripts from all colleges attended.

2. Volunteer or work in health settings

Most medical schools seek prospective students who have been exposed to physicians and patients in health-related settings. This demonstrates your knowledge and commitment to health science and to human service. Interviews often aggressively explore just how significant your involvement was.

3. Broaden your course selection

If possible, take classes that will expand your potential as a caring individual, community leader and physician.

4. Develop onsite advisors

Cultivate strong relationships with faculty who can advise and support you. These relationships will surely enrich your academic experience.

Professors can recommend courses and appropriate medical schools and write letters of recommendation. Professors might also invite you to work with them on projects or in their labs. Meet with professors and advisors at least three times each semester to discuss your aspirations, intellectual passions and extracurricular activities.

5. Prepare for the MCAT

Generally, performance on the MCAT mirrors SAT performance. Home study programs or more formalized MCAT review courses can improve performance.

6. Take the April MCAT if possible

The MCAT exam is offered twice each year, in April and August. An April MCAT allows scores to be delivered to AMCAS or AACOMAS in time for AMCAS and AACOMAS applications and affords the opportunity to repeat the test if necessary. The test should be taken 18 months prior to intended enrollment. For more information, contact MCAT at (319) 337-1357 or www.aamc.org.

7. Submit transcripts to AMCAS/AACOMAS

Transcripts require the greatest lead-time and should be requested, verified and sent prior to completion of your AMCAS, non-AMCAS or AACOMAS applications. Since official transcripts are accepted by AMCAS, AACOMAS and non-AMCAS schools beginning in mid March, you should request that each school you have attended send you a transcript.

Check each transcript for accuracy and then ask each school to send a single, official transcript to AMCAS or AACOMAS and an official transcript to each of your non-AMCAS participating schools.

Applications for AMCAS and AACOMAS are generally available April 1st and processed beginning June 1st. For information regarding application to allopathic medical schools, contact AMCAS at (202) 828-0600 or www.aamc.org. Application information regarding non-AMCAS schools must be obtained directly from these schools. For information regarding application to osteopathic medical schools, contact AACOMAS at (301) 968-4190 or www.aacom.org.

8. Submit applications early to optimize your chances

Early applications are associated with higher acceptance rates and greater likelihood of landing interviews. Submit applications as soon as possible and include your scores, transcripts, personal essay and letters of recommendation. Maintain records of all your applications.

9. Monitor application submission

Track the arrival of your applications to ensure their completeness and their receipt by each school to which you are applying. To assume safe delivery is to court disappointment. You must be your own best advocate in the application process.

The Admissions Committee and Its Function

In most medical schools, the Admissions Committee is comprised of 15 or more members of the general faculty, as well as representatives from the medical student body. The Dean of Admissions usually chairs the committee and he or she reports directly to the Medical School Dean. The committee first evaluates students by reviewing their credentials and letters of recommendation. Committee members also conduct interviews and submit written evaluations of interviewees. The entire committee discusses each candidate's application, with the interviewer often commenting on his or her impressions. During committee meetings, all members evaluate interviewed students and participate in the voting. Meetings are usually held weekly from early fall through the end of spring.

The File

The Admissions office maintains a file on each applicant. This file includes your AMCAS, AACOMAS, or non-AMCAS school application, your science and non-science GPA, grades from all transcripts, a list of the schools you have attended, all MCAT scores, letters of recommendation and your personal statement. In addition, your file may contain notations of support from phone contacts made in your behalf, and records of all written, verbal, and onsite inquiries you have made regarding your admission to the school.

The Personal Essay

The personal essay is the only truly personal statement you make prior to your interview. Use the essay to sell yourself. An effective essay will distinguish you from all other candidates, most of whom will have credentials nearly identical to your own. Some counsel:

Do

1. Catch the reader's attention from your first sentence. Skilled journalists know the power of a short, compelling lead. Keep your reader's attention with a well-organized, concise personal essay. A strong close will further convince your audience that it is in their best interest to interview you.

2. Describe specific accomplishments, giving the reader a well-focused and articulate view of who you are, your interests, experience and history.

3. In presenting your many achievements, do so within the context of gratitude for the opportunity rather than as a testimonial to your greatness or conquests.

4. Explain information in your application that might be viewed negatively by an admissions committee. This includes course failures, withdrawals, low MCAT scores, or unusual personal circumstances.

5. Focus on honest, concrete, original, biographical information. Use your own voice. If you do quote someone, make sure the quote is highly relevant and invigorates your message. Hackneyed quotes, no; fresh, witty, wise and pertinent, yes.

6. Make your essay visually inviting to read. Revise carefully for correct punctuation, spelling and grammar. Have others critique the essay for accuracy, clarity and style.

Don't

1. Criticize your school, departments or teachers. Stay positive.

2. Discuss controversial or argumentative views. Sell you.

3. Try to make too many points. You have one page to convey two to three messages. Provide evidence that will convince your reader that you are a winning candidate who will make the school and the reader proud. Lead the reader to this conclusion but don't state this conclusion yourself.

Transcripts

AMCAS and AACOMAS will provide you with a Transcript Matching Form. Obtain copies of transcripts for all undergraduate schools you have attended by January of your junior year. Once you have checked these for accuracy, have the registrars send official transcripts to AMCAS, AACOMAS and non-AMCAS schools. Complete the Academic Record portion of your AMCAS, AACOMAS or non-AMCAS application and send the application. Note that the Transcript Matching Form must accompany each transcript.

Chronology

1. Request and verify accuracy of transcripts from all schools attended.
2. Have each college send official transcripts and send Transcript Matching Forms to AMCAS, AACOMAS and non-AMCAS medical schools.
3. Expect notification of receipt of transcripts from AMCAS, AACOMAS and non-AMCAS medical schools two to three weeks after requesting that these be sent.
4. Obtain AMCAS, AACOMAS and non-AMCAS application forms.
5. Complete and copy forms for your records.
6. Send completed AMCAS, AACOMAS and non-AMCAS application forms with fees.

7. Expect notification of receipt of your application from AMCAS, AACOMAS and non-AMCAS medical schools two to three weeks after you send these.
8. Pay individual medical schools' requested application fees.
9. Send mid-year grades directly to schools.

The Purpose of the Interview

The interview provides the medical school with an opportunity to learn more about applicants. It also allows the medical school to promote its own unique features. By its nature, the interview is primarily subjective. It provides useful information that actively supplements the objective information in your application.

In most cases, the interview is structured to be non-confrontational, supportive and open. Most experienced interviewers concentrate on lowering the stress level rather than raising it, and expect the applicants to be relaxed and to be themselves. Within this open setting, the applicants are provided enough time to thoughtfully answer questions.

The institution seeks women and men with outstanding intellectual and personal qualifications. The admissions committee works to select a group of individuals who are diverse in backgrounds, training and talents, yet will function well together as a class.

Interviews help the committee identify a cohesive group of highly qualified individuals.

Qualifications Evaluated

Objective (GPA, MCAT) and subjective (recommendations, personal essay, interview) criteria help the admissions committee evaluate your application. These objective and subjective tools reveal your:

1. Personality
2. Maturity and honesty
3. Interpersonal skills
4. Communication skills
5. Motivation and commitment to practice medicine
6. Leadership qualities
7. Humanistic, social, and ethical concerns
8. Depth and breadth of knowledge
9. Critical thinking and coping skills
10. Creativity and original thinking

Committee Assessment

Generally, the interviewer is asked to dictate a report as soon as possible after the interview. Most evaluations are written in the interviewer's narrative style. The interviewer is asked to create a synopsis of the interview with his or her impressions. Often, the report will include interesting highlights that have been gleaned from the application folder. Most institutions grade interviews and merge interview scores with scores for MCATs, GPA, and letters of recommendation. The summation of these four scores creates a composite score. Then, candidates are ranked as outstanding, excellent, very good, good or average. If an applicant belongs to a special category, such as under-represented minority or alumni, he or she generally competes only against those within that category.

A formal presentation of the candidate before the entire committee occurs a week or two after the interview. Objective scores of GPA, both science and non-science, MCATs, and grades for letters of recommendation and interviews are presented to the committee. The interviewer is often asked to summarize the candidate and this provides an opportunity to promote the student's candidacy, reinforcing unique strengths and providing explanation for any weaknesses in the application. A full discussion ensues with questions directed to the interviewer. Finally, a consensus is reached whether the student should be accepted or denied admission.

Protocol for Tracking Status of Application

Most medical schools emphasize the integrity of the admissions process. The interviewer acts as an agent of the committee, and the decision whether to admit an applicant is a committee decision. All inquiries and communications that follow your interview should be directed to the admissions office. Do not attempt to contact the interviewer or Dean of Admissions directly or through agents for yourself. The Dean of Admissions will contact you when a decision is made.

One caveat: often students withhold all communications with the admissions office for fear of "bothering them." In some medical schools, the number of oral and written contacts with the admissions office are tracked as a reflection of your interest. You should always write the Dean of Admissions and your interviewer a thank you note following your interview. You may also check the status of your application from time to time and express your continued interest in the school.

10 Common Mistakes

1. Inadequate preparation for MCAT exams
MCAT performance mirrors SAT performance. If you are an average standardized test taker, consider an MCAT review course.

2. Late application
Submit applications early. This requires excellent planning and coordination of transcripts, MCAT's, recommendations, and applications. Ideally, you should begin planning two years before you intend to enroll.

3. Poor performance in core sciences

To be competitive, A's and B's in core sciences are generally required. An occasional C gets by, especially if accompanied by excellent MCAT's. Repeat core courses where you earned a C or below to demonstrate your mastery of the subject matter.

4. Lack of volunteer or health service experience

It has become a general expectation that candidates will pursue experiences that evince growth as a caring, service-oriented individual in the field of health care. This experience demonstrates your commitment to a life of medicine.

5. Poor choice of references

A single poor reference, even subtly stated, can send an application off track. Nurture relationships with future references early. Carefully assess the level of an individual's support for you. Consider choosing those who have already demonstrated concrete support for you through grades or other forms of recognition.

6. Poor personal essay

Write a clear, concise, well-organized and interesting statement. Check its grammar, punctuation, spelling and clarity. Seek qualified or expert critique and revise accordingly.

7. Failure to monitor application status

The application process is complex and requires sequential coordinated actions. Ensure that your completed application materials are submitted and confirm their receipt by July or August.

8. Inadequate research of school

Some of the 144 medical schools will ideally suit your personality, interests and talents; others will not. Thoroughly research medical colleges by reviewing literature, visiting campuses and conferring with pre-medical advisers, alumni and current medical students. Also consider factors such as in-state versus out-of-state admission rates.

9. Inadequate preparation for your interview

Although the interview commonly carries a quarter of the decision weight, and can actually collapse an otherwise qualified applicant, many students continue to "wing it." Careful research, preparation and performance are a must. The cardinal sins: appearing arrogant or disinterested.

10. Lack of post-interview follow through

In some schools, all verbal, written and physical contacts are captured in your application file. A thank you note to the Dean of Admissions and your interviewer is always appreciated. Gratitude is a becoming attitude in everyone, and a thank you letter leaves a favorable impression on the people who may accept you. Occasional respectful contacts to check on the status of your application are generally received as an expression of continued interest.

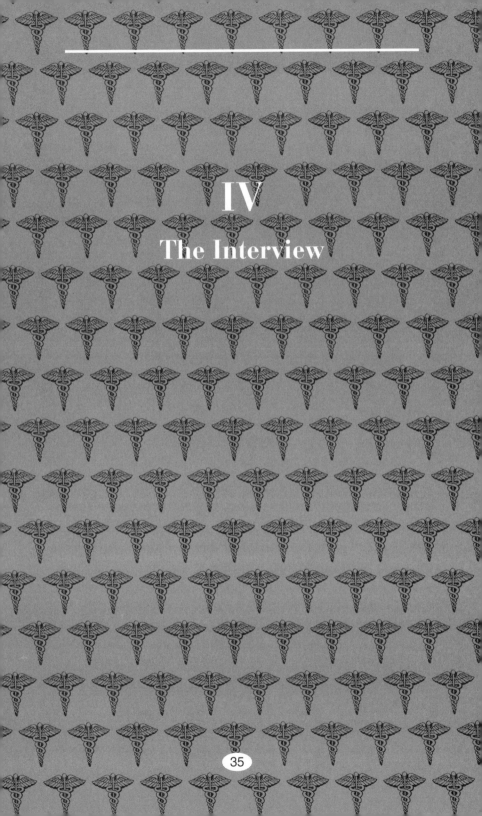

IV
The Interview

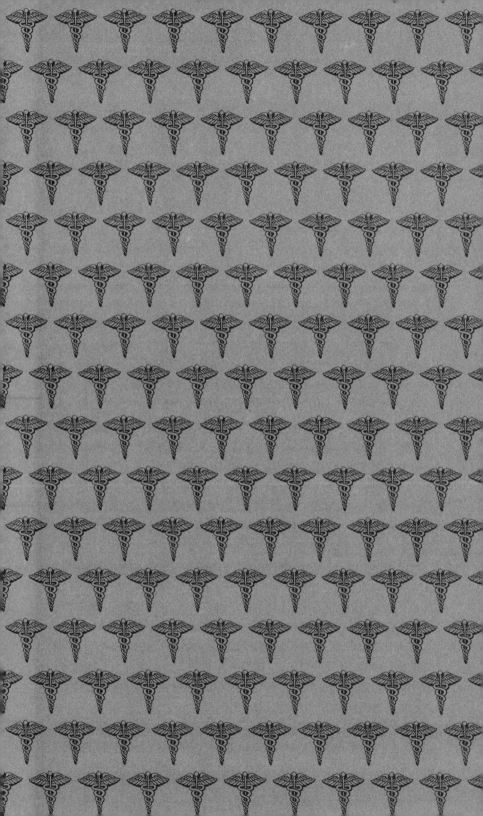

IV   The Interview

A Familiar Format

The most frequent type of interaction between two individuals is an interview with one individual soliciting information and the other providing it. Regard the medical school interview as an exchange of information. Since you were young, you have been approached and have approached others to obtain information. An interview also allows people to develop a relationship and an impression of one other. The interview is a most flexible format that can be highly individualized. It can move forward in a prearranged manner or adapt and pursue unexpected lines of inquiry. Thorough preparation lets you seize advantage of this format. Be prepared to provide accurate and comprehensive information while keeping it positive.

Preparation for the Interview

To assure a successful interview, prepare. Think of yourself as a reporter assigned an important issue to investigate. You need a clear understanding of the organization and individuals who will be interviewing you, and the message and image you intend to convey. Review the school's catalogue and other sources of information.

1. **Conduct the following self-inventory before your interview:**
- What is your objective?
- What is your message and how does it support your objective?
- Who is your audience?
- What do you know about this institution, its people, its curriculum and its culture?
- What do they know about you?
- Have you reviewed your own application?
- What within your application makes you uncomfortable?
- What do you hope they won't ask you and how will you answer when they do?
- Where and when is the interview?
- Have you made adequate arrangements for lodging?
- Have you allotted extra time so that you can arrive at your interview relaxed and on time?

2. **Interview Questions to Expect**
   Here are questions commonly asked during medical school interviews. Be prepared to answer each:
- What do you believe in?
- What do you care about?
- How does that caring express itself?
- How did you investigate a career in medicine?
- What made you decide to pursue a career in medicine?
- What is your favorite type of teaching style?
- What branch of medicine most interests you?

- Who knows you the best in this world?
- How would that person describe you, and what advice have they provided you?
- What teamwork experiences have you had?
- Who are your heroes?
- What are your strengths and weaknesses?
- What skills have you developed outside the classroom?
- Where do you see yourself in 10 years?
- What is the greatest obstacle you have had to overcome?
- What issues confront medicine today?
- What has been your greatest achievement?
- What person, past or present, would you most like to meet?
- What have you read recently in the press about health care?
- What makes you a better applicant than others?
- Why do you want to become a physician?
- How would you express your concern for a child needing an amputation?
- How do you relax?
- What is your biggest concern about entering medical school?
- Describe your best teacher and what made her or him unique.
- Describe an experience you had helping others.
- What was the last book you read?
- Describe an experience where you were misjudged.
- What has been your favorite non-science course and why?

- Who are your senators, congressmen, governor?
- What was your most difficult or demoralizing experience?
- What is the difference between sympathy and empathy?
- Is there anything you want to brag about or that you need to explain?
- If you are accepted to multiple schools, how will you make your decision?
- What is the toughest thing about being a patient?
- What type of criticism upsets you?
- Have you ever been a patient and, if so, can you reveal how that felt?
- How have your personal and volunteer experiences strengthened your goal to become a physician?
- What have been the strengths and weaknesses of your college preparation?
- Would you say you are most like your father or mother, and why?
- Why did you choose an osteopathic/allopathic school?
- What will you do next year if you don't get into medical school?
- Is this school your first choice?
- Why did you apply to this medical school?
- Is there anything I haven't asked you that you want to tell me?

The following subjects were covered in over two-thirds of the Class of 2006's medical school interviews:

- The source of your inspiration to pursue medicine
- Interpersonal qualities that will enhance your practice of medicine
- Specific qualities that lead to choice of this medical school
- Qualities that will insure your success as a medical school student and physician
- Interest in generalist versus specialist fields

The following topics are commonly raised regarding medical ethics:
- Privacy
- Children's rights
- Rights of the handicapped
- Rights of the terminally ill
- Rights of defective newborns
- Organ donation
- Care of the mentally handicapped
- Care of the elderly
- Determination of death
- Physician's responsibility for societal health

3. Physical Appearance

Physical appearance creates a first impression and impacts how you are perceived. Present yourself in a personable and professional manner. Some dress for success tips:
- Dress conservatively. Men should wear a suit or a blazer and neatly pressed pants with a dress shirt and simple tie. Women should wear a suit or solid dress.

- Women should avoid distracting or flashy jewelry.
- Jackets should be free of lapel pins.
- Remove bulky items from pockets.
- Collar and tie should be straight. Scarves should be in place.
- Avoid half-glasses or light-sensitive ones that conceal your eyes.

4. Body Language

Physicians are expected to be skilled communicators whose facial expressions and hand gestures carry their message. Your body language is closely observed by a physician interviewer. The following gestures convey aplomb, sincerity and interest:

- Make eye contact while you are listening.
- Sit erect but not stiff, leaning slightly forward.
- Use normal conversational hand movements to underscore your message.
- Listen intently to all questions and responses from the interviewer.

Avoid the following:

- Fidgeting or nervous gestures
- Inappropriate smiling or laughter
- Tightly grasping the arms of a chair or your hands in a prayer gesture
- Tightening and loosening your facial muscles
- Unnaturally straight, rigid posture
- Wandering eyes, paticularly when you are addressed or speaking

Interview Recommendations

1. There is no consistency from one interviewer to the next. Styles and approaches vary. Expect anything.

2. Most interviews are open and non-combative. Approach the interview with optimism.

3. Honesty is key.

4. Be prepared for questions regarding weaknesses or discrepancies in your application.

5. Don't list any honors, research projects, or volunteer experiences in your application that you will be unable to support as real and significant.

6. Ask questions if you have real ones about the school.

7. Read the school catalogue prior to the interview.

8. Do not ask what your chances are.

9. Do not get upset if the interviewer is late.

10. Allow the interviewer to interrupt you, but don't interrupt the interviewer.

11. Elaborate; don't dominate conversation.

12. Know your application file better than the interviewer (excluding your letters of recommendation).

13. Don't ask questions about your letters of recommendation if you have waived rights to see them.

14. Know something about the city you are visiting, even if only from that day's local newspaper or the taxi driver.

15. Don't try to second-guess the interviewer.

16. Avoid slang terms.

17. Be courteous and considerate toward all office staff.

18. If you know a student or faculty member personally, feel free to weave this naturally into the conversation, identifying her or him as a source of guidance and advice.

19. If this school is your first choice, state it. If not, explain your first choice if asked, and present this school as your second, if this is accurate.

20. If your choice of this school is tied to a fiancee's or spouse's choice, state it. Most schools are sympathetic to couples.

Optimal Arrival for the Interview

A thoroughly planned arrival tips the odds in your favor. If the interview is not in your immediate area, come the day before and stay overnight in a hotel or at a friend's home. Be sure that the accommodations are adequate for a good night's sleep and grooming the following morning. If possible, preview the physical site where the interview will take place. If you have the interview room number, arrive early to familiarize yourself with the location. Seeing the site with its physical arrangement avoids any sense of surprise that might shake your confidence during the interview. Awaken that morning with plenty of extra time so that you can properly groom, eat, and arrive with time to spare. Use the bathroom prior to the interview to check your clothes and your smile in the mirror.

Review the following quick tips for success:

1. Be honest

2. Be professional

3. Think fast but speak slowly

4. Be human and interesting

5. Smile. Believe in yourself and you will transfer this belief to your interviewer.

Relaxation Techniques

Most candidates experience appropriate anxiety as they approach their interview. Remember that confidence is earned and you only acquire it by meeting challenges in a positive, determined spirit. If nervous in the final hour, try the following:

- Walk around the block, let your muscles relax, your eyes wander and b-r-e-a-t-h-e. Whistle. Sing.
- Stretch your arms, legs, torso and facial muscles.
- Think of treasured or humorous memories. Smile or laugh.
- Breathe deeply, counting for a number of seconds, then hold your breath the equivalent number of seconds and finally exhale for as long as you can. Repeat this, each time lengthening the breath, the hold and the exhalation.
- If you are in a room awaiting the interviewer's arrival, practice deep breathing and alternately tense and relax your muscles, head to toe.
- Acknowledge that even seasoned professionals experience some stage fright. If controlled, this energizes and enhances your performance.
- Remember to believe in the very best within you.

The Appearance

The interview begins when the interviewer enters the room. Rise and greet the interviewer professionally with a firm handshake and a smile. Express your pleasure and gratitude for the opportunity to interview at this medical school. While the interviewer will take the lead and ask the questions, it's important to keep in mind that you mutually own this interview. Ideally, you will enjoy an interpersonal exchange that connects and enriches you both.

Some key points:

1. Be personal and professional
Doctors may begin somewhat formally. Interviews often begin tensely and gradually yield to a warmer, more relaxed atmosphere. Mirror the mood of the interviewer and stay positive.

2. Stay on message
You should have in mind two or three points that you wish to convey during the interview. Seek opportunities early to introduce and reinforce these points.

3. Practice active listening
Listen carefully to questions posed. Clarify any inquiry or information that is unclear before you respond.

4. Control the pace
When nervous, most people speak too quickly. A controlled, slower pace shows a contemplative, more self-possessed candidate.

5. Monitor your body language

Be aware that your body is a powerful communication tool.

6. Stay alert, polite, poised

Skilled interviewers will attempt to relax you so that you will be honest and spontaneous with them. Their goal is to get to know the real you. This is your goal as well. Remember, though, that you need to maintain a polished, professional demeanor.

7. Maintain respectful, interested eye contact

Use eye contact as you would when fully engaged in an interesting conversation with a friend.

8. Affirm the positive

If asked a question that provides an opportunity to voice something you think is important, restate the question during your response. You might even reveal that you are glad the interviewer broached the subject.

9. Proceed mindfully

Stay within the bounds of a professional interview. The interviewer is not a trusted confidante or close friend. Rather, the interviewer is appraising your personal qualities and communication skills. Humor can jeopardize your candidacy. You needn't be stiff or refrain from smiling. Just save your favorite joke for a more appropriate audience.

10. Enjoy the interview and learn from it

At the end of your meeting, you will know more about the interviewer, yourself, and this prospective medical school. Your performance will be improved by an attitude that emphasizes exploration rather than fear.

Tough Questions...

Foresee tough question or ones that come from left field. Try to provide a reasonable and informed response. It is not so much what you say, but how you say it. Some counsel:

1. Acknowledge that this is a difficult question. This shows that you are listening and gives you a few moments to prepare a reasoned, balanced response.

2. Demonstrate concern and thoughtfulness in your response and maintain a moderate voice.

3. Above all, don't take a tough question personally. Often, an interviewer poses difficult questions to test your resilience.

4. Do not argue or become defensive. The last thing you want to do is dispute the interviewer.

5. Modulate your body language. You may want to verbally retaliate, but your body should do just the opposite. This softens the impact of the trying question and demonstrates your equilibirium.

6. Segue to a more favorable message. While addressing the question, relate it to a subject that contains some of the major messages you want to convey. Candidates who can turn the tables so diplomatically prove their mettle and grace.

7. Don't be overwhelmed. Your whole life is not on the line. If one hard question can undo you, you may not be able to withstand the rigors of this demanding profession.

8. Conclude your response on an amicable, positive note.

Post Interview Self-Evaluation

Now that you have made it through the interview, your work isn't over. Breathe, walk, eat, and then sit down within an hour of your interview and answer the following questions:

1. Did I stay on message?
2. Was I in control?
3. Did I tell the truth and avoid exaggeration?
4. Was I calm and did I pace myself well?
5. Did I anticipate the questions?
6. Did I present a positive, professional image?
7. Did I listen carefully?
8. Was I a credible candidate?
9. Could I have done better and how?
10. What did I learn?

There's always something you could have done a little bit better. Through conscientious introspection, you will continually develop your interpersonal skills.

Summary of Interview Advice

In summation:

1. Be Prepared: Have something to say. Say it with style, force and intelligence.

2. Be Human: Medicine requires excellent communication and people skills, composure and poise. During your interview, demonstrate your maturity, thoughtfulness and sensitivity.

3. Be Yourself: Physicians regularly practice reading people's overt and covert responses. Be yourself, trust in your preparation and in human nature and learn from your experience.

Good luck!

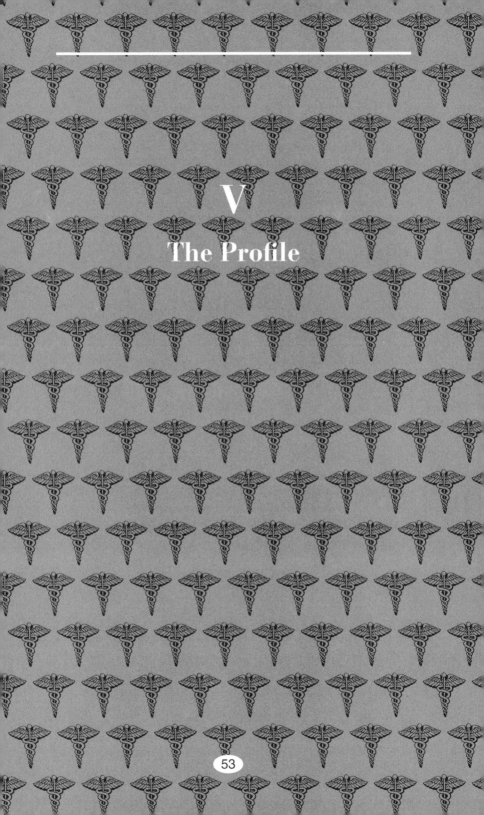

V

The Profile

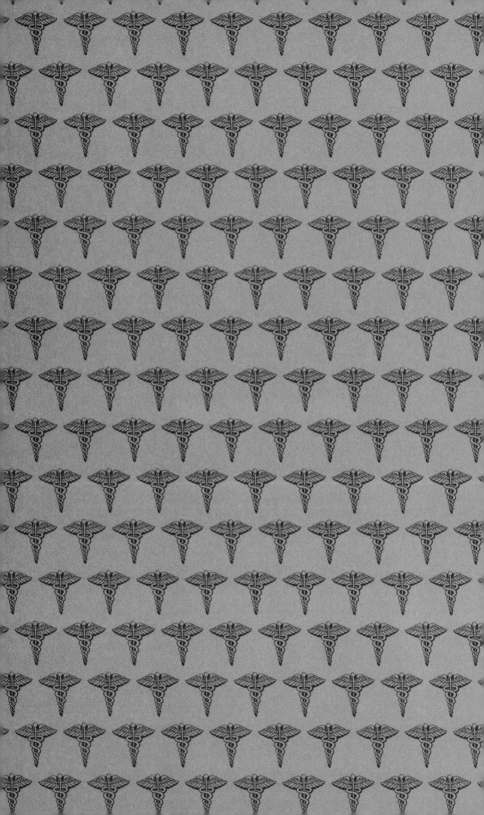

V   The Profile

The Class of 2006

A Profile of the Class of 2006 (in round figures):

Allopathic
- 125 schools
- 34,859 applicants
- 17,456 entrants
- 50% acceptance
- 47.5% women
- 10.6% under-represented minorities
- 11.6 applications/applicant
- 59% Public/41% Private

Average Admission Scores

MCAT
VR	9.4
PS	9.7
BS	9.8

GPA
Sciences	3.44
Total	3.49

Osteopathic

- 19 schools
- 6,898 applicants
- 2,927 entrants
- 42% acceptance
- 36.6% women
- 7.6% under-represented minorities
- 5.7 applications/applicant
- 22% Public/78% Private

Average Entrant Scores

MCAT
VR	8.1
PS	8.2
BS	8.7

GPA
Sciences	3.36
Total	3.5

Medical Students' Beliefs:

A 1995 survey of matriculating medical students conducted by the Association of American Medical Colleges revealed the following beliefs:

1. Physicians will receive the same respect from society as they have in the past.
2. Opportunities to build a successful practice are always available to physicians who work hard.
3. Having interesting and intelligent colleagues is a major benefit of being a physician.
4. Everyone is entitled to receive adequate medical care regardless of his or her station in life.
5. Physicians have an opportunity to exercise greater influence on health promotion and disease prevention.
6. Physicians have an obligation to care for a reasonable number of patients who will be unable to pay a doctor's bill.
7. Technological advances will make being a doctor in the future more fulfilling.
8. Physicians have an ethical duty to treat patients with infectious diseases even if there is a risk of contracting the disease.
9. Equal access to medical care remains a problem in the United States.
10. Medicine will not be as financially rewarding in the future as in the past.

Top five reasons for choosing medicine:
1. Opportunity to make a difference.
2. Educate patients about health.
3. Intellectual challenge and critical thinking.
4. Contact with patients.
5. Exercise social responsibility.

Top five reasons students chose a particular medical school:
1. General reputation of school.
2. Geographic location.
3. Teaching methods of school.
4. School's curriculum.
5. Financial cost of attending/school's ability to place in residency programs.

CLASS OF 2006

Medical School	Class Size	% In-State Pupils	% Women	Resident Tuition	Non-Resident Tuition
Alabama					
University of Alabama*	160	88	39	7,564	22,692
University of South Alabama	64	86	38	7,700	15,400
Arizona					
Arizona College of Medicine§	125	24	40	25,000	25,000
University of Arizona	100	100	48	9,600	N/A
Arkansas					
University of Arkansas	146	97	40	10,080	20,160
California					
University of California Davis*	93	99	50	0	10,704
University of California Irvine*	94	100	44	0	10,704
University of California Los Angeles*	121	79	42	0	10,244
University of California San Diego*	121	94	42	0	10,704
University of California San Francisco*	141	82	60	0	10,704
Loma Linda University	163	48	41	28,015	28,015
University of Southern California	160	87	43	34,130	34,130
Stanford University	86	47	50	31,497	31,497
Touro University College of Medicine§*	125	50	43	25,000	25,000
Western University of the Health Sciences§	176	78	45	28,010	28,010
Colorado					
University of Colorado	127	86	46	11,966	59,597
Connecticut					
University of Connecticut*	76	82	52	10,040	22,840
Yale University	100	10	49	30,900	30,900
Washington, DC					
George Washington University	154	1	48	33,800	33,800
Georgetown University	170	2	44	30,838	30,838
Howard University	105	7	49	18,070	18,070

CLASS OF 2006

Medical School	Class Size	% In-State Pupils	% Women	Resident Tuition	Non-Resident Tuition
Florida					
Nova Southeastern University COM§	180	55	33	21,245	26,395
University of Florida	97	99	46	10,931	30,855
University of Miami	142	95	50	27,233	35,670
University of South Florida	100	100	35	10,930	30,820
Georgia					
Emory University	112	35	41	29,548	29,548
Medical College of Georgia	180	88	31	7,340	29,358
Mercer University	58	100	37	23,620	29,358
Morehouse School of Medicine	41	68	60	20,160	20,160
Hawaii					
University of Hawaii	62	90	47	13,632	27,336
Illinois					
Chicago College of Medicine§	160	50	40	24,185	29,374
University of Chicago Pritzker	104	38	50	27,120	27,120
Chicago Medical School	193	23	40	35,678	35,673
University of Illinois	317	82	40	17,664	41,420
Loyola University of Chicago	130	50	45	30,500	30,500
Northwestern University	170	31	44	32,805	32,805
Rush Medical College	120	86	44	29,616	29,616
Southern Illinois University	71	99	43	13,346	40,038
Indiana					
Indiana University	280	91	39	15,300	33,238
Iowa					
University of Iowa	150	69	40	14,504	32,972
Des Moines University of Osteopathic Medicine and Surgery§*	204	25	40	25,475	25,475
Kansas					
University of Kansas	175	84	40	10,600	24,812

CLASS OF 2006

Medical School	Class Size	% In-State Pupils	% Women	Resident Tuition	Non-Resident Tuition
Kentucky					
University of Kentucky	96	92	48	11,089	25,803
University of Louisville	141	88	48	12,424	31,046
Pikeville College§ School of Osteopathic Medicine (PCSOM)	65	63	47	24,255	24,255
Louisiana					
Louisiana State – New Orleans	166	99	42	8,856	23,004
Louisiana State – Shreveport	100	100	33	8,581	22,729
Tulane University	154	21	45	31,830	31,830
Maine					
University of New England COM§	117	75	60	29,100	29,100
Maryland					
Johns Hopkins University*	118	6	47	28,100	28,100
University of Maryland	137	82	51	13,954	26,701
Uniformed Service University	167	7	23	0	0
Massachusetts					
Boston University	154	19	45	36,530	36,530
Harvard Medical School	167	10	47	29,000	29,000
University of Massachusetts	100	100	51	8,352	N/A
Tufts University	168	29	41	37,875	37,875
Michigan					
College of Osteopathic Medicine§*	125	90	46	17,448	37,248
Michigan State University	96	87	52	16,416	36,219
University of Michigan	170	49	41	18,538	28,898
Wayne State University	256	89	40	14,203	29,557
Minnesota					
Mayo Medical School	42	33	52	20,500	20,500
University of Minnesota – Duluth	54	94	51	21,615	40,156
University of Minnesota – Minneapolis	165	72	46	21,165	40,156

CLASS OF 2006

Medical School	Class Size	% In-State Pupils	% Women	Resident Tuition	Non-Resident Tuition
Mississippi					
University of Mississippi	100	100	36	6,938	13,298
Missouri					
Kirksville COM§	158	13	27	26,450	26,450
University of Health Science COM§	225	17	37	29,990	29,990
University of Missouri – Columbia	95	98	48	15,458	30,060
University of Missouri – Kansas City	111	87	62	22,752	46,099
St. Louis University	153	37	46	33,300	33,300
Washington University	120	5	48	34,280	34,280
Nebraska					
Creighton University	115	14	44	31,326	31,326
University of Nebraska	110	85	45	13,870	29,505
Nevada					
University of Nevada	52	90	40	8,417	24,669
New Hampshire					
Dartmouth Medical School	81	8	50	28,655	28,655
New Jersey					
University of Med & Dent of NJ	170	100*	42	17,362	27,164
		*all out-of-state students qualified for in-state residency			
UMDNJ					
– Robert Wood Johnson	142	87	48	17,362	27,164
UMDNJ – School of OM§	85	80	45	17,362	27,169
New Mexico					
University of New Mexico	75	97	54	9,015	25,843

CLASS OF 2006

Medical School	Class Size	% In-State Pupils	% Women	Resident Tuition	Non-Resident Tuition
New York					
Albany Medical College	131	40	54	33,925	33,954
Albert Einstein College of Medicine	180	49	52	31,450	31,450
Columbia University	150	16	44	32,454	32,454
Cornell University Weill Medical College	101	45	54	27,650	27,650
Mt. Sinai School of Medicine	105	38	49	25,250	25,250
New York COMs*	260	83	48	26,775	26,775
New York Medical College	188	32	56	31,320	31,320
New York University*	160	44	40	24,950	24,950
University of Rochester	100	41	51	29,100	29,000
State University of NY – Downstate	160	93	44	12,840	24,940
University of Buffalo	135	96	58	12,840	24,940
State University of NY – Stony Brook	102	99	45	12,840	24,940
State University of NY – Syracuse	156	92	45	12,840	24,940
North Carolina					
Duke University*	98	11	49	28,566	28,566
East Carolina University Brody	72	100	50	2,951	23,618
University of NC Chapel Hill	160	89	49	5,123	28,126
Wake Forrest University School of Medicine	108	50	41	29,640	29,640
North Dakota					
University of North Dakota	57	46	35	12,538	33,474
Ohio					
Case Western Reserve	144	59	43	33,735	33,735
University of Cincinnati	154	76	38	14,782	26,385
Medical College of Ohio	140	79	30	13,068	29,640
Northeastern Ohio University	117	100	44	13,806	27,612
Ohio State University	210	76	39	13,848	35,853
Ohio University COMs	110	86	43	16,452	23,976
Wright State University	90	92	55	12,066	17,088

CLASS OF 2006

Medical School	Class Size	% In-State Pupils	% Women	Resident Tuition	Non-Resident Tuition
Oklahoma					
Oklahoma State University COM§	88	85	38	11,557	30,144
University of Oklahoma	149	98	41	10,698	26,439
Oregon					
Oregon Health Sciences	101	67	45	15,888	33,483
Pennsylvania					
Lake Erie COM§	212	64	35	22,720	23,720
Jefferson Medical College	223	48	40	30,979	30,979
Medical College of PA Hahnemann	237	35	47	30,305	30,305
Pennsylvania State University	124	44	44	21,936	30,496
University of Pennsylvania	148	27	43	31,940	31,940
Philadelphia COM§	250	68	45	28,500	28,500
University of Pittsburgh	147	41	48	24,100	32,542
Temple University	210	67	39	25,740	31,378
Puerto Rico					
Universidad Central del Caribe*	60	78	45	17,000	24,000
Ponce School of Medicine	63	84	39	17,835	26,597
University of Puerto Rico	116	100	50	5,000	10,500
Rhode Island					
Brown University	69	16	56	29,608	29,608
South Carolina					
Medical University of South Carolina*	141	96	42	3,756	12,069
University of South Carolina	70	86	40	10,350	29,890
South Dakota					
University of South Dakota	50	92	46	10,826	25,932

CLASS OF 2006

Medical School	Class Size	% In-State Pupils	% Women	Resident Tuition	Non-Resident Tuition
Tennessee					
East Tennessee State University	60	98	44	13,082	26,666
Meharry Medical College*	80	27	48	23,208	23,208
University of Tennessee	165	92	59	27,602	27,602
Vanderbilt University	104	7	39	27,325	27,325
Texas					
Baylor College of Medicine	168	73	52	6,550	19,650
Texas A&M	68	96	98	6,550	19,650
Texas College of OM§	111	90	45	6,550	19,650
Texas Tech University	120	97	28	7,325	20,425
University of Texas – Dallas	204	87	35	6,920	20,020
University of Texas – Galveston	205	93	41	6,550	19,650
University of Texas – Houston	204	97	41	7,450	20,550
University of Texas – San Antonio	208	94	49	6,550	19,650
Utah					
University of Utah	102	73	32	10,695	20,247
Vermont					
University of Vermont	95	32	53	20,520	35,900
Virginia					
Eastern Virginia Medical School	105	81	43	16,000	29,500
Virginia Commonwealth University	180	62	40	11,062	28,360
University of Virginia	139	60	42	14,154	26,654
Washington					
University of Washington	179	91	50	10,143	25,668
West Virginia					
Marshall University	48	88	41	10,080	26,010
West Virginia School of OM§	75	68	51	14,206	35,158
West Virginia University	90	92	39	8,728	20,958

CLASS OF 2006

Medical School	Class Size	% In-State Pupils	% Women	Resident Tuition	Non-Resident Tuition
Wisconsin					
Medical College of Wisconsin	204	58	38	19,604	29,695
University of Wisconsin	150	84	47	18,566	28,068

* The tuition figures above do not include student fees. Student fees range from $500 to $1500 for most schools. Schools marked with an asterisk have student fees ranging from $2500 to $7000.

Contact schools directly to confirm current student tuition and fees.

§ Denotes osteopathic medical school.

N/A Denotes not applicable.

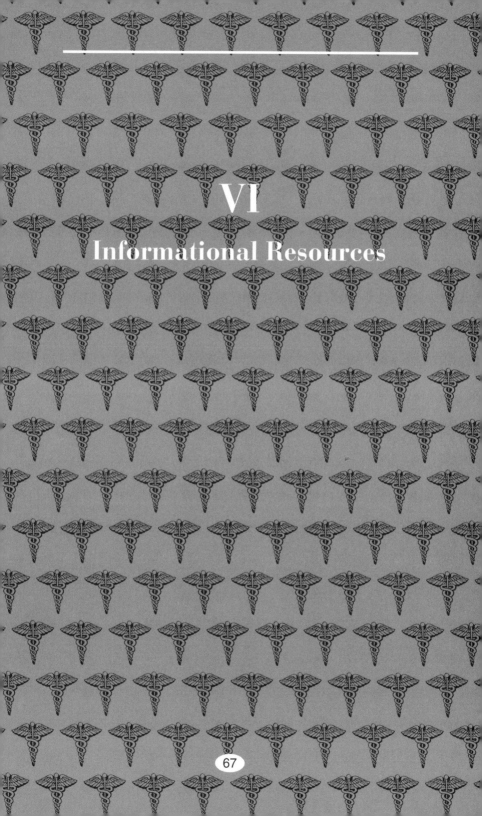

VI
Informational Resources

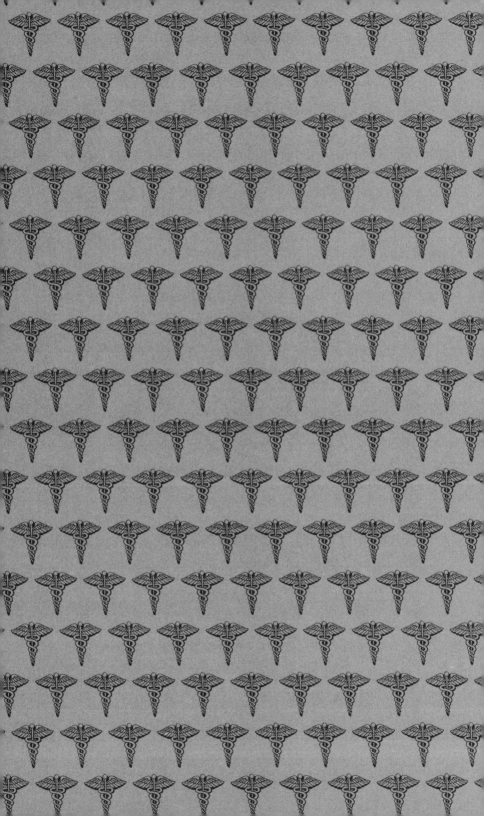

VI Informational Resources

Print Information

These printed resources may be useful supplements to your educational and financial planning:

1. *The Student Guide, 2003-2004.* Department of Education. Free. EDPubs. PO Box 1398, Jessup, MD 20794-1398 (877) 433-7827

2. *Dollars for College: The Quick Guide to Scholarships, Fellowships, Loans, and Other Financial Aid Programs for Medicine, Dentistry and Related Fields.* $6.95 plus shipping and handling. Garrett Park Press, P.O. Box 190, Garrett Park, MD 20896; (301) 946-2553; ISBN: 1-880774-15-1

3. *Financial Planning and Management Manual for U.S. Medical Students.* Association of American Medical Colleges. $7.50 plus shipping and handling. Association of American Medical Colleges, Publications Department, 2450 N Street, NW, Washington, DC 20037; (202) 828-0416

4. *Cass & Birnbaum Guide to American Colleges.* 17th edition – out of print. M., and Cass-Liepmann, J., eds., $19.95 paperback. Harper/Collins Publishers, Inc., Publications Department, 1000 Keystone Industrial Park, Scranton, PA 18512; (570) 941-1500; ISBN: 0062734040

5. *The College Board Guide to 150 Popular Majors.* Item #004000 $16.00, plus $4.00 postage and sales tax where applicable. Used copies available through amazon.com for $10.50 plus shipping and handling. College Board Publications, 45 Columbus Avenue, New York, NY 10023-0886; (212) 713-8000

6. *The College Cost and Financial Aid Handbook, 2003 ed.* Item #006674. $22.95, plus sales tax where applicable. Revised annually each September. College Board Publications, 45 Columbus Ave., New York, NY 10023-0886; (212) 713-8000*

7. *The College Handbook.* Item #006658. $26.95, plus sales tax where applicable. Revised annually each September. College Board Publications, 45 Columbus Ave., New York, NY 10023-0886; (212) 713-8000*

8. *Index of Majors and Graduate Degrees.* Item #006666. $22.95, plus sales tax where applicable. Revised annually each September. College Board Publications, 45 Columbus Ave., New York, NY 10023-0886; 212-713-8000*

* NOTE: A package set containing the items described in #s 6, 7 and 8 above is available at a cost of $52.00 and may be ordered under item #990787 by contacting College Board Publications, either by mail or by phoning (212) 713-8000.

9. *Financial Aids for Higher Education.* 1995. 17th ed. Santamaria, O. $80.63 plus sales tax where applicable and shipping and handling. McGraw-Hill, 860 Taylor Station Road, Blacklick, OH 43004; (800) 262-4729; ISBN: 06-97-241513

10. *Meeting College Costs, 2002.* Item #00607. $13.95, plus sales tax where applicable. College Board Publications, 45 Columbus Ave., New York, NY 10023-0886; (212) 713-8000

11. *Need a Lift? College Financial Aid Handbook.* Item #75207.2. $3.00 prepaid, plus sales tax where applicable and shipping and handling. The American Legion Emblem Sales, P.O. Box 1050, Indianapolis, IN 46206; (888) 453-4466

12. *Medical School Admission Requirements 2003-2004.* $25.00 plus shipping. Association of American Medical Colleges, 2450 N Street, NW, Washington, DC 20037; (202) 828-0416

13. *Health Professions Career & Education Directory, 2002-2003 edition.* $65.00, non-members; $55.00 members, plus $8.95 for handling and shipping. Order No. OP-417502BQH. American Medical Association, P.O. Box 930876, Atlanta, GA 31193-0876; Attn: Order Department; (800) 621-8335

14. *270 Ways To Put Your Talent To Work in the Health Field.* Single copy, $18.00, non-members; $15.00, members plus shipping and handling. National Health Council, 1730 M Street, NW, Suite 500, Washington, DC 20036; (202) 785-3910

15. *Medical Student Financial Aid Resource Guide 2000.* Free to AMA members. American Medical Association, Medical Student Services, 515 North State Street, Chicago, IL 60610; (312) 464-5000

Health Careers Information

These professional associations provide information useful to health professionals:

1. Association of American Medical Colleges
   2450 N Street, NW
   Washington, DC 120037
   (202) 828-0416
   web site: www.aamc.org

2. American Association of Colleges of Osteopathic Medicine
   Suite 310
   5550 Friendship Boulevard
   Chevy Chase, MD 20815
   (301) 968-4100
   web site: www.aacom.org

3. American Association of Colleges of Pharmacy
   1426 Prince Street
   Alexandria, VA 22314-2841
   (703) 739-2330
   web site: www.aacp.org

4. American Association of Colleges of Podiatric Medicine
   Suite 322
   1350 Piccard Drive
   Rockville, MD 20850-4307
   (800) 443-3514
   web site: www.adea.org

5. American Dental Education Association
   Suite 600
   1625 Massachusetts Avenue, NW
   Washington, DC 20036-2212
   (202) 667-9433
   web site: www.adea.org

6. Association of American Veterinary Medical Colleges
   Suite 710
   1101 Vermont Avenue, NW
   Washington, DC 20005-3521
   (202) 371-9195
   web site: www.aavmc.org

7. Association of Schools and Colleges of Optometry
   Suite 510
   6110 Executive Boulevard
   Rockville, MD 20852
   (301) 231-5944
   web site: www.opted.org

8. Association of Schools of Public Health
   1101 15th Street, NW
   Suite 910
   Washington, DC 20005
   (202) 296-1099
   fax: (202) 296-1252
   web site: www.asph.org

9. National Association of Advisors to the Health Professions
   P.O. Box 1518
   Champaign, IL 61824
   (217) 355-0063
   web site: www.naahp.org

10. Alpha Epsilon Delta
    National Headquarters
    James Madison University
    MSC 4307,
    701 Carrier Drive
    Harrisonburg, VA 22807
    (540) 568-2594
    email: aed@jmu.edu #
    web site: www.jmu.edu/orgs/nationalaed

Electronic Information:

www.positiveprofiles.com – Pfizer Medical Humanities Initiative; offers email access to medical schools nationwide, publications, scholarship information, physician profiles, inspirational stories, links to other resources.

www.aamc.org – offers information on America's 125 allopathic medical schools.

www.aacom.org – offers information on America's 19 osteopathic medical schools.

www.ama-assn.org/go/becominganmd – offers information on becoming an MD.

www.ama-assn.org/ama/pub/category/2322.html – offers information on careers in allied health professions.

www.kaplan.com – offers MCAT preparation and information.

www.review.com – offers MCAT preparation and information.

www.naahp.org – National Association of Advisors to the Health Professions

www.asph.org – Association of Schools of Public Health

www.jmu.edu/orgs/nationalaed – national medical honor society, Alpha Epsilon Delta

www.aacp.org – American Association of Colleges of Pharmacy

www.aacpm.org – American Association of Colleges of Podiatric Medicine

www.adea.org – American Dental Education Association

www.aavmc.org – Association of American Veterinary Medical Colleges

www.opted.org – Association of Schools and Colleges of Optometry

Medical Science Information:

ama-assn.org – The American Medical Association

cmwf.org – The Commonwealth Fund

drkoop.com – Dr. Koop

jama.com – The Journal of the American Medical Association

mayohealth.org – Mayo Clinic Health Oasis

nhionline.net – National Health Information

nlm.nih.gov – National Institutes of Health

nejm.org – The New England Journal of Medicine

pfizer.com – Pfizer Inc.

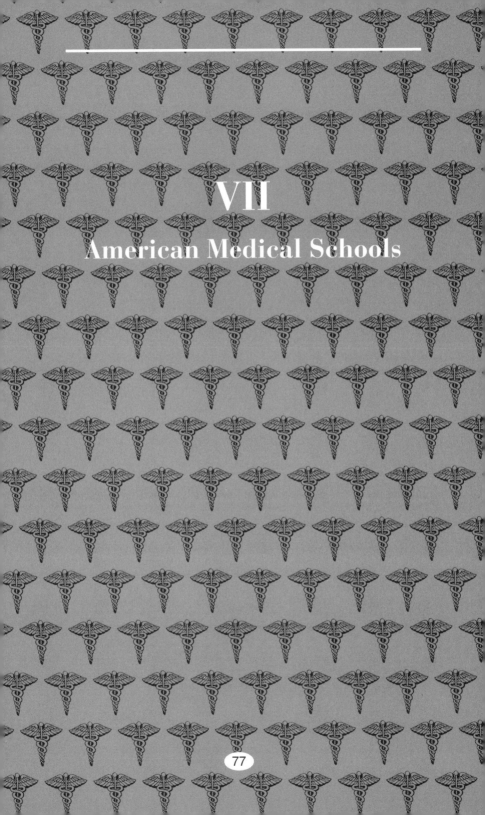

VII
American Medical Schools

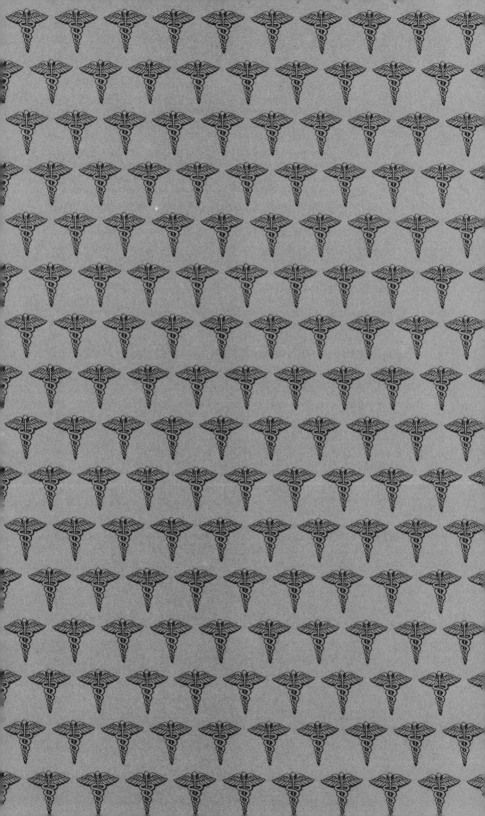

VII American Medical Schools

Admissions Contact Person & Address

ALABAMA

University of Alabama School of
Medicine
Dr. Nathan Smith
Assistant Dean for Admissions
Office of Medical Student
Services/Admissions VH P100
Birmingham, AL 35294-0019
205-934-2330

University of South Alabama
College of Medicine
Mr. Mark Scott
Director for Admissions
Office of Admissions 241 CSAB
Mobile, AL 36688-0002
334-460-7176

ARIZONA

University of Arizona College of
Medicine
Dr. Christopher Leadem
Admissions Office, Rm 2209
P.O. Box 245075
Tucson, AZ 85724-5075
520-626-6214

Arizona College of Osteopathic
Medicine§
Jim Walter
Director of Admissions
19555 N. 59th Avenue
Glendale, AZ 85308
888-247-9277

ARKANSAS

University of Arkansas for Medical
Sciences College of Medicine
Tom G. South
Director of Admissions
4301 W. Markham St., Slot 551
Little Rock, AK 72205-7199
501-686-5354

CALIFORNIA

University of California, Davis
School of Medicine
Dr. Edward Dagang
Associate Dean for Student Affairs
Admissions Office
1 Shield Avenue
Davis, CA 95616
530-752-2717

University of California, Irvine
College of Medicine
Gayle Pierce
Director of Admissions
P.O. Box 4089
Medical Education Bldg., 802
Irvine, CA 92697-5981
949-824-5388

University of California, Los
Angeles
UCLA School of Medicine
Dr. Neil Parker
Associate Dean for Admissions
P.O. Box 957035
Office of Student Affairs
12-105 Center for Health Sciences
Los Angeles, CA 90095-7035
310-825-6081

University of California, San Diego
School of Medicine
Dr. Robert Resnik
Associate Dean for Admissions
0621/Medical Teaching Facility
9500 Gilman Drive
LaJolla, CA 92093-0621
858-534-3880

University of California, San Francisco
School of Medicine
Dr. Henry Ralston
Associate Dean of Admissions
521 Parnass Avenue
C-200, Box 0408
San Francisco, CA 94143-0408
415-476-4044

Loma Linda University
School of Medicine
Dr. John Thorn
Associate Dean for Admissions
11234 Anderson Street, MC A-522
Loma Linda, CA 92350
909-558-4467

University of Southern California
School of Medicine
Joe Allen
Dean of Admissions
1975 Zonal Avenue (KAM 100-C)
Los Angeles, CA 90089
323-442-2552

Touro University College of
Osteopathic Medicine§
Dr. Donald Haight
Director of Admissions
832 Walnut Street
Quarters C
Vallejo, CA 94592
888-887-7336

Stanford University School of
Medicine
Dr. Gabriel Garcia
Associate Dean for MD Admissions
251 Campus Drive
MSOB Room 341
Stanford, CA 94305-5404
650-723-6861

Western University of the Health
Sciences/
College of Osteopathic Medicine of
the Pacific§
Susan Hanson
Director of Admissions
309 East 2nd Street
Pomona, CA 91766-1854
909-469-5335

COLORADO

University of Colorado
School of Medicine
Dr. Maureen J. Garrity
Associate Dean for Admissions
4200 E. Ninth Avenue, C-297
Denver, CO 80262
303-315-7361

CONNECTICUT

University of Connecticut School
of Medicine
Keat Sanford
Assistant Dean
263 Farmington Ave., Rm AG-062
Farmington, CT 06030-3906
860-679-4306

Yale University School of Medicine
Dr. Thomas L. Lentz
Associate Dean – Admissions
Office of Admissions
367 Cedar Street
New Haven, CT 06510
203-785-2643

WASHINGTON, DC

George Washington University
School of Medicine and Health
Sciences
Dr. Brian McGrath
Associate Dean for Admissions
2300 Eye Street, NW, Room 615
Washington, DC 20037
202-994-3506

Georgetown University School
of Medicine
Eugene T. Ford
Director of Admissions
Office of Admissions
3900 Reservoir Road, NW
Washington, DC 20007
202-687-1154

Howard University College of
Medicine
Ann Finney
Admissions Officer
520 W Street, NW
Washington, DC 20059
202-806-6270

FLORIDA

Nova Southeastern University
College of Osteopathic Medicine§
Marla Frohlinger
Vice Chancellor – Student Affairs
3200 S. University Drive
Fort Lauderdale, FL 33328
954-262-1101

University of Florida College of
Medicine
Dr. Ira Gessner
Chair, Medical Selection Committee
Box 100216
J. Hillis Miller Health Center
Gainesville, FL 32610
352-392-4569

University of Miami School of
Medicine
Dr. R.E. Hinkley
Associate Dean for Admissions
P.O. Box 016159
Miami, FL 33101
305-243-6791

University of South Florida
College of Medicine
Dr. John Ackerman
Assistant Dean of Admissions
Box 3, 12901 Bruce B. Downs Blvd.
Tampa, FL 33612-4799
813-974-2229

GEORGIA

Emory University School of
Medicine
Dr. J. William Eley
Associate Dean/Director of
Admissions
Woodruff Health Sciences Building
1440 Clifton Road, NE, Room 115
Atlanta, GA 30322
404-727-5660

Medical College of Georgia
School of Medicine
Dr. Mason Thompson
Associate Dean for Admissions
AA-2040
Augusta, GA 30912-4760
706-721-3186

Mercer University School of
Medicine
Dr. A. Peter Eveland
Associate Dean for Admissions
Office of Admissions & Student
Affairs
1550 College Street
Macon, GA 31207-0001
478-301-2542

Morehouse School of Medicine
Dr. Angela Franklin
Associate Dean – Student Affairs/
Admissions
720 Westview Drive, SW
Atlanta, GA 30310-1495
404-752-1650

HAWAII

University of Hawaii
John A. Burns School of Medicine
Dr. Satoru Izutsu
Associate Dean/Chair, Adm Com
1960 East-West Road
Honolulu, HI 96822
808-956-5505

ILLINOIS

Chicago College of Osteopathic
Medicine§
Raeleru Brower
Director of Admissions
555 31st Street
Downer's Grove, IL 60515
800-458-6253

University of Chicago
Pritzker School of Medicine
Sylvia Robertson
Assistant Dean of Admissions
924 E. 57th Street, BLSC 104
Chicago, IL 60637-5416
773-702-1937

Finch University of Health
Sciences
Chicago Medical School
Kristine A. Jones
Director of Admissions
3333 Green Bay Road
N. Chicago, IL 60064
847-578-3206

University of Illinois College of
Medicine
Dr. Jorge A. Girotti
Associate Dean and Director of
Admissions
Room 165 CME M/C 783
808 S. Wood Street
Chicago, IL 60612-7302
312-996-5635

Loyola University Chicago
Stritch School of Medicine
LaDonna E. Norstrom
Assistant Dean, Admissions
Office of Admissions
2160 S. First Avenue
Building 120, Room 200
Maywood, IL 60153
708-216-3229

Northwestern University
Medical School
Dolores Brown
Associate Dean for Admissions
Morton 1-606
303 E. Chicago Avenue
Chicago, IL 60611-3008
312-503-8206

Rush Medical College of Rush
University
Jan L. Schmidt
Director of Admissions
524 Academic Facility
600 S. Paulina Street
Chicago, IL 60612
312-942-6913

Southern Illinois University
School of Medicine
Erin L. Graham
Director of Admissions
Office of Student Affairs
P.O. Box 19624
Springfield, IL 62794-9624
217-524-6013

INDIANA

Indiana University School of
Medicine
Lynde J. Means MD
Director of Admissions
Fesler Hall 213
1120 South Drive
Indianapolis, IN 46202-5113
317-274-3772

IOWA

University of Iowa College of
Medicine
Catherine Solow
Director of Admissions
100 Medicine Administration
Building
Iowa City, IA 52242-1101
319-335-8052

Des Moines University
Osteopathic Medical Center§
Becky Grissom
Director of Admissions &
Enrollment Development
3200 Grand Avenue
Des Moines, IA 50312
800-240-2767 (ext. 1450)

KANSAS

University of Kansas School of
Medicine
Sandra J. McCurdy, MEd
Assistant Dean for Admissions
3901 Rainbow Boulevard
Kansas City, KS 66160-7301
913-588-5245

KENTUCKY

University of Kentucky College of
Medicine
Dr. Carol L. Elam
Assistant Dean for Admissions
Admissions Room MN-102
Office of Education
800 Rose Street
Lexington, KY 40536-0298
859-323-6161

University of Louisville School
of Medicine
Stephen F. Wheeler, MD
Associate Dean of Admissions
Health Sciences Center
323 East Chestnut Street
Louisville, KY 40202-3866
502-852-5193

Pikeville College School of
Osteopathic Medicine (PCSOM)§
Dr. Jeanne Kietzer
Director of Admissions
147 Sycamore Street
Pikeville, KY 41501-1194
606-218-5406

LOUISIANA

Louisiana State University
School of Medicine in New Orleans
Dr. Sam G. McClugage
Asst. Dean for Admissions
1901 Perdido Street, Box P3-4
New Orleans, LA 70112-1393
504-568-6262

Louisiana State University
School of Medicine in Shreveport
Dr. F. Scott Kennedy
Assistant Dean for Student
Admissions
1501 Kings Highway
Shreveport, LA 71130-3932
318-675-5190

Tulane University School of
Medicine
Dr. Joseph C. Pisano
Associate Dean
1430 Tulane Avenue, SL67
New Orleans, LA 70112-2699
504-588-5187

MAINE

University of New England
College of Osteopathic Medicine§
Patricia Cribby
Asst. Director Medical Admissions
11 Hills Beach Road
Biddeford, ME 04005
800-477-4UNE

MARYLAND

Johns Hopkins University
School of Medicine
James Weiss, MD
Associate Dean – Admissions
720 Rutland Avenue
Baltimore, MD 21205-2196
410-955-3182

University of Maryland
School of Medicine
Dr. Milford M. Foxwell, Jr.
Associate Dean for Admissions
Room 1-005, 655 W. Baltimore St.
Baltimore, MD 21201
410-706-7478

Uniformed Services University of
the Health Sciences
F. Edward Hebert School of
Medicine
Peter J. Stavish, LTC, MS, USA (Ret)
Assistant Dean for Admissions &
Academic Records
Admissions Office, Room A-1041
4301 Jones Bridge Road
Bethesda, MD 20814-4799
301-295-3101

MASSACHUSETTS

Boston University School of
Medicine
Dr. John F. O'Connor
Associate Dean for Admissions
Building L, Room 124
715 Albany Street
Boston, MA 02118
617-638-4630

Harvard Medical School
Dr. Jules L. Dienstag
Faculty Associate Dean for
Admissions
25 Shattuck Street, Suite A-210
Boston, MA 02115-6092
617-432-1550

University of Massachusetts
Medical School
Dr. Jon Paraskos
Associate Dean for Admissions
55 Lake Avenue, N
Worcester, MA 01655
508-856-2323

Tufts University School of
Medicine
Thomas M. Slavin
Director of Admissions
136 Harrison Avenue
Boston, MA 02111
617-636-6571

MICHIGAN

College of Osteopathic Medicine[§]
Kathie Schaefer
Director of Admissions
C110 East Fee Hall
Michigan State University
East Lansing, MI 48824-1316
517-353-7740

Michigan State University
College of Human Medicine
Christine L. Shafer, MD
Asst. Dean, Admissions
A-239 Life Sciences
Michigan State University
East Lansing, MI 48824-1317
517-353-9620

University of Michigan Medical
School
Dr. Joyce Wahr
Dean – Admissions/Financial Aid
D4303, Medical Science I Building
1301 Catherine
Ann Arbor, MI 48109-0611
734-764-6317

Wayne State University School
of Medicine
Dr. Joseph Dogariu
Assistant Dean for Admissions
540 E. Canfield
Detroit, MI 48201
313-577-1466

MINNESOTA

Mayo Medical School
Dr. Thomas R. Viggiano
Associate Dean for Student Affairs
200 First Street, SW
Rochester, MN 55905
507-284-3671

University of Minnesota – Duluth
School of Medicine
Dr. Lillian Repesh
Assoc. Dean for Admissions/
Student Affairs
Room 180
10 University Drive
Duluth, MN 55812
218-726-8511

University of Minnesota
Medical School – Minneapolis
Dr. Marilyn Becker
Associate Dean/Admissions
MMC – 293
420 Delaware Street, SE
Minneapolis, MN 55455-0310
612-626-1188

MISSISSIPPI

University of Mississippi School
of Medicine
Dr. Steven Case
Associate Dean – Admissions
2500 N. State Street
Jackson, MS 39216-4505
601-984-5010

MISSOURI

Kirksville College of Osteopathic
Medicine[§]
Lori A. Haxton
Director of Admissions
800 West Jefferson Street
Kirksville, MO 63501
660-626-2237

University of Health Sciences
College of Osteopathic Medicine[§]
Minnie G. Marrs
Admissions Director
1750 Independence Boulevard
Kansas City, MO 64106-1453
800-234-4847

University of Missouri –
Columbia School of Medicine
Judy Nolke
Admissions Coordinator
MA213-215,
Medical Science Building
One Hospital Drive
Columbia, MO 65212
573-882-2923

University of Missouri-Kansas City*
School of Medicine
Mary Anne Morgenegg
Admissions Cordinator
Counsel on Selection
2411 Holmes
Kansas City, MO 64108
816-235-1870

St. Louis University School
of Medicine
Dr. James Willmore
Associate Dean of Admissions
1402 S. Grand Boulevard
St. Louis, MO 63104
314-577-8205

Washington University School
of Medicine
Dr. W. Edwin Dodson
Associate Dean for Admissions
660 S. Euclid Avenue, #8107
St. Louis, MO 63110
314-362-6858

NEBRASKA

Creighton University School
of Medicine
Henry Nipper, MD
Assistant Dean
Medical School Admissions
2500 California Plaza
Omaha, NE 68178
402-280-2798

University of Nebraska College
of Medicine
Dr. Jeffrey W. Hill
Assoc. Dean of Admissions and
Student Affairs
Office of Admissions
986585 Nebraska Medical Center
Omaha, NE 68198-6585
402-559-6140

NEVADA

University of Nevada School
of Medicine
Dr. Jerry R. May
Associate Dean for Admissions
Mail Stop 357
Reno, NV 89557
775-784-6063

NEW HAMPSHIRE

Dartmouth Medical School
Andrew G. Welch
Director of Admissions
3 Rope Ferry Road
Hanover, NH 03755-1404
603-650-1505

NEW JERSEY

University of Medicine and
Dentistry of NJ
New Jersey Medical School
Dr. George F. Heinrich
Assistant Dean for Admissions
185 S. Orange Avenue
Newark, NJ 07103
973-972-4631

University of Medicine and
Dentistry of NJ
Robert Wood Johnson Medical
School
Dr. David Seiden
Associate Dean for Admissions
Admissions Office
675 Hoes Lane
Piscataway, NJ 08854
732-235-4576

University of Medicine and
Dentistry of New Jersey
School of Osteopathic Medicine[§]
Warren Wallace, Ed.D.
Associate Dean of Admissions
and Student Affairs
Office of Admissions, Suite 162
1st Floor Academic Center
One Medical Center Drive
Stratford, NJ 08084
856-566-7050

NEW MEXICO

University of New Mexico
School of Medicine
Dr. Roger Radloff
Interim Assistant Dean for
Admissions
Basic Medical Science Bldg,
Room 107
Albuquerque, NM 87131-5166
505-272-3814

NEW YORK

Albany Medical College
Sara J. Kremer
Director of Admissions
Office of Admissions, A-3
47 New Scotland Avenue
Albany, NY 12208
518-262-5521

Albert Einstein College of
Medicine of Yeshiva University
Noreen Kerrigan
Assistant Dean for Student Adm
Jack & Pearl Resnick Campus
1300 Morris Park Avenue
Bronx, NY 10461
718-430-2106

Columbia University[*]
College of Physicians and
Surgeons
Dr. Andrew G. Frantz
Associate Dean – Admissions
Admissions Office, Room 1-416
PO Box 41
630 West 168th Street
New York, NY 10032
212-305-3595

Cornell University Weill Medical
College
Dr. Charles Bardes
Associate Dean/Chair, Admissions
Committee
Room 104
445 East 69th Street
New York, NY 10021
212-746-1067

Mt. Sinai School of Medicine of
the City University of NY
Dr. Alex Stagnaro-Green
Dean for Student Affairs
Annenberg Building, Room 5-12
1 Gustave L. Levy Pl., Box 1255
New York, NY 10029
212-241-6691

New York Institute of Technology
of the New York College of
Osteopathic Medicine[§]
Michael J. Schaefer
Director of Admissions
PO Box 8000
Old Westbury, NY 11568
516-626-6947

New York Medical College
Dr. Fern Juster
Associate Dean/Chair, Admissions
Committee
Sunshine Cottage
Valhalla, NY 10595
914-594-4507

New York University School of
Medicine*
Raymond J. Brienza
Assistant Dean for Admissions
PO Box 1924
New York, NY 10016
212-263-5290

University of Rochester
School of Medicine and Dentistry
Pat Samuelson
Director of Admissions
Medical Center
601 Elmwood Avenue, Box 601-A
Rochester, NY 14642
585-275-4539

State University of New York
Health Science Center at Brooklyn
College of Medicine
Thomas Lo
Director of Admissions
450 Clarkson Avenue, Box 60M
Brooklyn, NY 11203
718-270-2446

University of Buffalo
School of Medicine and
Biomedical Sciences
Dr. Thomas J. Guttuso
Assistant Dean, Admissions
Room 45, Biomed. Ed. Building
3435 Main Street
Buffalo, NY 14214-3013
716-829-3466

SUNY at Stony Brook School
of Medicine
Health Sciences Center
Jack Fuhrer
Associate Dean/Director for
Admissions – Level 4
Stony Brook, NY 11794-8434
631-444-2113

State University of New York
Health Science Center at Syracuse
College of Medicine
Ronald Wolk
Associate Dean, Student Affairs
155 Elizabeth Blackwell Street
Syracuse, NY 13210
315-464-4570

NORTH CAROLINA

Brody School of Medicine at
East Carolina University
Dr. James G. Peden Jr.
Associate Dean for Admissions
Office of Admission, AD-52
Greenville, NC 27858-4354
252-816-2202

Duke University School of
Medicine
Dr. Brenda E. Armstrong
Associate Dean, Director of
Admissions
PO Box 3710
Durham, NC 27710
919-684-2985

Wake Forrest University
School of Medicine
Bowman Gray Campus
Dr. Lewis H. Nelson, III
Associate Dean for Admissions
Medical Center Boulevard
Winston-Salem, NC 27157-1090
336-716-4264

University of North Carolina at
Chapel Hill
School of Medicine
Dr. Axalla Hoole
Associate Dean – Admissions
121 MacNider Hall
Chapel Hill, NC 27599-7000
919-962-8331

NORTH DAKOTA

University of North Dakota*
School of Medicine
Judy L. DeMers
Associate Dean, Student Affairs &
Admissions
501 N. Columbia Road, Box 9037
Grand Forks, ND 58202-9037
701-777-4221

OHIO

Case Western Reserve University
School of Medicine
Dr. Albert C. Kirby
Associate Dean for Admissions
10900 Euclid Avenue
Cleveland, OH 44106-4920
216-368-3450

University of Cincinnati
College of Medicine
Dr. J. Robert Suriano
Associate Dean for Admissions
PO Box 670552
Cincinnati, OH 45267-0552
513-558-7314

Medical College of Ohio
Dr. Mary Ann Myers
Associate Dean for Admissions
3045 Arlington Avenue
Toledo, OH 43614-5805
419-381-4229

Northeastern Ohio Universities
College of Medicine
Dr. Bonnie Jones
Associate Dean for Admissions
PO Box 95
4209 State Rt 44
Rootstown, OH 44272-0095
330-325-6270

Ohio State University College
of Medicine
Dr. Mark A. Notestine, Ph.D.
Assistant Dean & Director of
Admissions
270 Meiling Hall
370 W. Ninth Avenue
Columbus, OH 43210-1238
614-292-7137

Ohio University College of
Osteopathic Medicine[§]
James P. Artis, Ph.D.
Director of Admissions
102 Grosvenor Hall
Athens, OH 45701-2979
740-593-4313

Wright State University
School of Medicine
Dr. Paul G. Carlson
Associate Dean for Admissions
PO Box 1751
Dayton, OH 45401
937-775-2934

OKLAHOMA

Oklahoma State University
College of Osteopathic Medicine[§]
Bonnie Laster
Associate Director of Admissions
and Recruitment
1111 W. 17th Street
Tulsa, OK 74107
918-582-1972

University of Oklahoma College
of Medicine
Dotty Shaw Killam
Director for Admissions
BMSB – 374
PO Box 26901
Oklahoma City, OK 73190
405-271-2331

OREGON

Oregon Health Sciences University
School of Medicine
Vicki Fields
Administrative Director,
Education/Student Affairs
3181 SW Sam Jackson Park Road
Portland, OR 97201
503-494-2998

PENNSYLVANIA

Lake Erie College of Osteopathic
Medicine§
Elaine Morse
Admissions Coordinator
1858 W. Grandview Boulevard
Erie, PA 16509
814-866-6641

Jefferson Medical College
Dr. Clara Callahan
Associate Dean for Admissions
1015 Walnut Street, Suite 110
Philadelphia, PA 19107
215-955-6983

MCP Hahnemann University
School of Medicine
Dr. Alan Tunkel
Assoc Dean of Admissions
2900 Queen Lane
Philadelphia, PA 19129
215-991-8202

Pennsylvania State University
College of Medicine
Dr. Dwight Davis
Associate Dean for Admissions
Suite C 1505
500 University
PO Box 850
Hershey, PA 17033-0850
717-531-8755

Philadelphia College of
Osteopathic Medicine§
Carol A. Fox
Assistant Dean for Admissions
4170 City Avenue
Philadelphia, PA 19131
215-871-6100

University of Pennsylvania
School of Medicine
Gaye W. Sheffler
Director of Admissions
Office of Admissions/Financial
Aid
Edward J. Stemmler Hall, Ste 100
Philadelphia, PA 19104-6056
215-898-8001

University of Pittsburgh
School of Medicine
Dr. Edward I. Curtiss
Associate Dean of Admissions
518 Scaife Hall
3550 Terrace Street
Pittsburgh, PA 15261
412-648-9891

Temple University School of
Medicine
Audrey B. Uknis, MD
Assistant Dean for Admissions
Suite 305 Student Faculty Center
3340 N. Broad Street
Philadelphia, PA 19140
215-707-3656

PUERTO RICO

Universidad Central del Caribe
School of Medicine
Dr. Helen Rosa
Dean of Medicine
Office of Admissions
PO Box 60-327
Bayamon, Puerto Rico 00960-6032
787-740-1611

Ponce School of Medicine
Dr. Carmen M. Mercado
Assistant Dean of Admissions
PO Box 7004
Ponce, Puerto Rico 00732-7004
787-840-2511

University of Puerto Rico
School of Medicine
Rita Aponte-Rodriguez
Director of Admissions
PO Box 365067
San Juan, Puerto Rico 00936-5067
787-758-2525

RHODE ISLAND

Brown University School of
Medicine*
Dr. Stephen R. Smith
Associate Dean for Medical
Education
Box G-A212
97 Waterman Street
Providence, RI 02912-9706
401-863-2149

SOUTH CAROLINA

Medical University of South
Carolina College of Medicine
Dr. Paul Underwood
Chair for Admissions
41 Bee Street
PO Box 250203
Charleston, SC 29425
843-792-3281

University of South Carolina
School of Medicine
Dr. Richard Hoppmann
Associate Dean for Student
Programs
Columbia, SC 29208
803-733-3325

SOUTH DAKOTA

University of South Dakota
School of Medicine
Dr. Paul Bunger
Dean – Admissions
Lee Medical Building, Room 105
414 E. Clark Street
Vermillion, SD 57069-2390
605-677-5233

TENNESSEE

East Tennessee State University
James H. Quillen College of
Medicine
Edwin D. Taylor
Assistant Dean for Admissions
PO Box 70580
Johnson City, TN 37614-0580
423-439-4753

Meharry Medical College
School of Medicine
Allen Mosley
Director/Admissions and Records
1005 D.B. Todd Boulevard
Nashville, TN 37208
615-327-6223

University of Tennessee, Memphis
College of Medicine
Dr. Hershel P. Wall
Associate Dean for Admissions
790 Madison Avenue
Memphis, TN 38163-2166
901-448-5559

Vanderbilt University School of
Medicine
Pat Sagen
Director of Admissions Committee
209 Light Hall
Nashville, TN 37232-0685
615-322-2145

TEXAS

Baylor College of Medicine
Dr. Major Bradshaw
Dean of Medical Education
One Baylor Plaza, Room N104
Houston, TX 77030
713-798-4842

Texas A&M University Health
Sciences
Center College of Medicine*
Filomeno G. Maldonado
Dean of Admissions
159 Reynolds Medical Bldg.
College Station, TX 77843-1114
979-845-7744

Texas Tech University*
Health Sciences Center
School of Medicine
Dr. Bernell Dalley
Associate Dean, Education
Lubbock, TX 79430-6216
806-743-2297

Texas College of Osteopathic
Medicine§
Jane Anderson
Director Medical Student
Admissions
3500 Camp Bowie Blvd.
Fort Worth, TX 76107-2699
817-735-2204

University of Texas*
Southwestern Medical Center
at Dallas
Sandra L. Hofman, MD, PhD.
Chairman of Admissions
5323 Harry Hines Boulevard
Dallas, TX 75390-9162
214-648-5617

University of Texas*
Medical School at Galveston
Dr. Cecilia Romero
Associate Dean – Admissions/
Student Affairs at Interim
301 University Blvd.
Galveston, TX 77555-1317
409-772-3517

University of Texas*
Houston Medical School
Albert E. Gunn, Esq.
Associate Dean for Admissions
6431 Fannin
MSB 1.126
Houston, TX 77030
713-500-5116

University of Texas*
Medical School at San Antonio
Dr. Davis Jones
Dean of Admissions
7703 Floyd Curl Drive
San Antonio, TX 78229-3900
210-567-2665

UTAH

University of Utah School of
Medicine
Dr. Victoria E. Judd
Associate Dean, Admissions
30 North 1900 East #1C029
Salt Lake City, UT 84132
801-581-7498

VERMONT

University of Vermont College
of Medicine
Dr. Cathleen J. Gleeson
Director of Admissions
E-215 Given Building
Burlington, VT 05405-0068
802-656-2154

VIRGINIA

Eastern Virginia Medical School
of the Medical College of
Hampton Roads
Susan L. Castora
Director of Admissions
721 Fairfax Avenue
Norfolk, VA 23507-2000
757-446-5812

Virginia Commonwealth
University
Medical College of Virginia
School of Medicine
Cynthia M. Heldberg
Assoc. Dean for Admissions
MCV Station, Box 980565
Richmond, VA 23298-0565
804-828-9629

University of Virginia School of
Medicine
Dr. Beth A. Bailey
Dean of Admissions
Admissions Office, Box 800725
Charlotteville, VA 22908
434-924-5571

WASHINGTON

University of Washington
School of Medicine
Dr. Werner E. Sampson
Dean for Admissions
Health Sciences Center A-300
Box 356340
Seattle, WA 98195-6340
314-362-6858

WEST VIRGINIA

Marshall University School of
Medicine
Cynthia A. Warren
Director of Admissions
1600 Medical Center Drive
Suite 3400
Huntington, WV 25701-3655
304-691-1738

West Virginia School of
Osteopathic Medicine§
John N. Gorby
Director of Admissions
400 North Lee Street
Lewisburg, WV 24901
800-356-7836

West Virginia University
School of Medicine
Dr. David Morgan
Director of Admissions Committee
PO Box 9111
Morgantown, WV 26506-6009
304-293-3521

WISCONSIN

Medical College of Wisconsin
Sharon A. Carpenter
Director of Admissions
8701 Watertown Plank Road
Milwaukee, WI 53226
414-456-8246

University of Wisconsin Medical
School
Mikel Snow, PhD.
Associate Dean for Admissions
Medical Sciences Center
Room 1140
1300 University Avenue
Madison, WI 53706-1532
608-263-4925

* Denotes non-AMCAS allopathic
  medical school

§ Denotes osteopathic medical
  school

Personal Notes

Personal Notes

Personal Notes

Personal Notes